This is where reviewers'
reviews are presented.

There are none because there's no time to spend to get reviewers before going to print. Only you or another person who knows someone with Lyme may understand this.

It is my deep wish that you, a loved one, or a friend soon recovers from Lyme.

May it be soon.

Treating Lyme with Antabuse

an outline for healing

Treating Lyme with Antabuse

an outline for healing

Fonda Living

Stream of Wisdom Press
San Francisco

Published by
Stream of Wisdom Press, San Francisco, CA.

This book is available through Amazon.

Cover Design by Stream of Wisdom Press.
Graphics and editing by Sara Frucht.
Thank you to Sara and to our ghostwriter.

Library of Congress Cataloguing-In-Publication Data

Names: Fonda Living, Author
Title: Treating Lyme with Antabuse :
An outline for healing / Fonda Living.
Description: 1st edition. | San Francisco, CA:
Stream of Wisdom Press, 2022.
Identifiers: LCCN 202293457 | ISBN 9780998614540 (softcover)
Subjects: Lyme, Lyme Disease, Disulfiram, Antabuse, Medical Recovery, Health, Medicine, Healing

Classification: LCCN 2022935457

Softcover ISBN 978-0-9986145-4-0

e ISBN 978-0-9986145-0-2

10 9 8 7 6 5 4 3 2

First edition, March 2022

Printed in the United States of America

To you who suffer
every day with Lyme
Never knowing when it will end
Wondering whether you are
on the right treatment or if you
need to change it to something else
whether you can pay your bills
whether you can work.

To my family and friends
who supported me even when
some did not believe
I had Lyme.

To everyone around me who did not know day to day I was in a proverbial hand-to-hand combat in an attempt to overcome Lyme.

May everyone be healed.

CONTENTS

DISCLAIMER

The information provided in this book is not meant to replace the guidance of a licensed medical practitioner. Nothing contained herein is meant to diagnose or prescribe. No information herein is meant to be a substitute for consulting with your licensed medical physician. Statements in this book have not been evaluated by the FDA.

Disulfiram, also known as Antabuse, is not to be taken with alcohol or fermented products (see page 26).

ACKNOWLEDGEMENTS

To the doctors who treated me:

I can't say your names here. You may have helped me when you were not supposed to help me the way you did. Thank you for your kindness. I am in your debt.

Many of my organs and joints would have been harmed without the interventions to stop the spirochetes.

To Braco's Gaze, His Holiness the Dalai Lama's online teaching, Joel Osteen, Brad Yates EFT, the TCM Medical Clinic nearby, and to my friends and family, I appreciate you.

You saved me.

PREFACE

You don't know when it will ever end. For you, like everyone with Lyme, this is urgent. Maybe like me, you are hiding it from many of your friends.

Often Lyme cases are way worse than mine. Mine was hidden to everyone-- I could do everything and I was able to sleep normally, but still I had symptoms. These symptoms meant I had Lyme. It wasn't like a cold where if you were 97% better you could stop taking the remedy. I knew there could not be a single spirochete left or it would repopulate.

On 2/22/22 in a moment of synchronicity, I attended a Harvard webinar with Kris Newby producer of the documentary, Under the Skin, and award-winning journalist Brian Owens author of Lyme Disease in Canada.

Kris Newby and her husband contracted Lyme in 2002 while on Martha's Vineyard. She said it took 5 years, 10 doctors and $60,000 to finally get her disease under control. Kris produced the award-winnging documentary *Under the Skin* and her book *Bitten* has won three international book awards.

The award-winning documentary shows the harrowing pain of people infected with Lyme. It estimates the pandemic number of Lyme patients in the US eclipses the numbers of both those with HIV and breast cancer.

Since this is an emergency for everyone with Lyme, I am writing this book. Here's a story you may need to hear which is how I am on the way to recovering. May you too be on your way to recovering too. Just bring every ounce of your courage.

What is Lyme?
CDC cases and warnings

"Lyme disease is the most common vector-borne disease in the United States. Lyme disease is caused by the bacterium Borrelia burgdorferi, Bb, and rarely, Borrelia mayonii, Bm. It is transmitted to humans through the bite of infected blacklegged ticks. Typical symptoms include fever, headache, fatigue, and a characteristic skin rash called erythema migrans (EM) [The CDC left out sweats, chills, and migrating joint pain.] If left untreated, infection can spread to joints, the heart, and the nervous system. [The CDC left out: Infection to the heart called Lyme carditis might lead a patient to require a heart transplant.]

"Most recent estimates are of 476,000 new cases of Lyme in the US every year. Scientists estimate that two million people could suffer from post-treatment Lyme disease at the end of 2020. Lyme disease has also been found in 80 countries," according to the CDC website.

Who am I and why may you trust me?

I am a San Francisco Bay Area resident who has struggled with Lyme for over four years. I work in STEM type work when I'm on contract in my field. I have a meditation practice and I do what I can to help or enliven people.

I'm a friendly, warm, engaging person. I drive a Honda and used to drink Americanos. I like to hike and explore museums. In recent months, I went to the Pompei exhibit in the Legion of Honor and the teamLab exhibit at the Asian Art Museum.

I'm writing this book to save you from the challenges I experienced taking Disulfiram. If Disulfiram is what your Lyme-Aware Doctor suggests as treatment, I hope this book encourages you on your path.

Who wants to write a book about Lyme anyway except to encourage others?

When I knew I would recover

You need to hear this.

It was not long ago on a Friday, when I was driving home from a friend's house in Marin. It was late and I was tired.

As I was driving, I realized something for the first time-- I realized my body felt different, that it didn't seem to be having the usual spirochete biting symptoms.

Then an enormous faith and knowing came over me:

I realized I would recover from Lyme.

I was sure of it.

This was the first time I remember believing I would recover for sure.

The next day I realized I had all but recovered. I had not yet recovered, but I realized I would recover. I realized that I was essentially on my way to complete recovery.

I called a very good friend of mine, a doctor who knows my medical situation, but only believes in lab results.

"Hey, I have some good news to tell you".

"What?" She asked.

"I've all but recovered from Lyme--
I don't have the usual symptoms.
--Ah, but you don't even believe
I have Lyme without labs to prove it."

On the other end of the line she said, "Even though I don't believe it, I can celebrate that you don't have the usual symptoms".

Since this is an urgent matter for everyone with Lyme this means I am writing while I am still treating, while producing this book as quickly as possible.

There were times even shortly before I realized I would recover that I thought I would not make it. I thought my life was over and I almost gave up emotionally.

The symptoms would not stop. Meanwhile, to everyone I looked normal. And while I was, I wasn't.

I knew that Lyme could destroy my heart, brain, and other organs... that it was, as some said, worse than cancer and that an infection to the heart, called Lyme carditis, may even require a heart transplant.

I thought this ordeal would never end.

And then one day, I realized it would.

My Story

It was 2017. I was a very healthy person before any of this happened, taking only vitamins and occasionally over the counter medicine such as aspirin and Chinese medicine.

During that year's Thanksgiving, as in years past, I invited friends to go on a hike and share Thanksgiving dinner together.

We headed out to West Marin to Roy's Redwoods to hike.

We were 14 people strong that year. A troupe of three groups headed in all directions in brilliant streaming sunlight in those warm afternoon woods. I laughed as I searched for the stragglers still coming, knowing there were three other groups somewhere at large who could not agree on a hike together in those woods.

After our hike, we drove out to Point

Reyes Station where we shared a healthy turkey or faux turkey dinner, potatoes, gravy, yams, cranberry sauce and all the fixin's. We could hardly hear ourselves talking to each other in the place where we were merrily eating dinner.

COCO, the movie, was just out and after dinner we regrouped in a park. We realized it was getting too cold to stay outside, so we decided to go see COCO.

Then someone in our group who happened to be a doctor with long hair and a large brimmed hat felt something moving on the right side of her neck. She reached to get whatever it was with her fingers. It was a tick. She freaked. We were all shocked because not only did she have this long hair, she was wearing this huge brimmed hat. How did it get there we wondered considering all her protective covering.

That was the proverbial warning shot across the bow. We all knew we should check for ticks. We headed out to see COCO which was fabulous. We went home to our different lives after a great day of celebration.

It was some days after our trip in the woods, while I was working from home, I started to notice that my right hip was hurting. Somehow, I spotted the Erythema Migrans (EM), a bullseye mark on the skin which is what remains where the tick has dined. The EM was located on my back right hip just over the bikini line. The tick was not there, but had had its fill. The bullseye or EM the tick leaves is a calling card of sorts. It was 12.5 days after our trip in the woods, a serious amount of potential time for the tick to be attached and to leave its payload.

Today's doctors are generally limited by formulary, a treatment of three to four weeks of doxycycline for a Lyme tick bite. My doctor gave four weeks of doxcycline. It was way outside the short window in which doxycycline would be effective, which is during the first two or three days of a tick attachment. I begged them to think outside the box, and requested an intramuscular shot of Penicillin G, Bicillin LA right in the tick bite site. They refused. Two to three weeks after the doxcycline, I had an unusual sore throat, unlike any other I had had before. I was unable to stop it with Zinc and Vitamin C, or any other tricks up my sleeve including Qing Qi Hua Tan Wang or Andrographis.

At eight weeks, I had migrating joint pain from hip to knee and then opposite knee and hip, all around like a merry-go-round, another characteristic of Lyme.

Around that time what I call "pins and needles" or "bites from inside" swarmed as an attack from the inside. At first this was accompanied by sweats and chills.

The joint pain in my hip reached 8-9 out of 10 level according to my notes. I used cat's claw, otoba bark, stevia, serrapeptase, houttunia, reservatrol, Vitamin A, EFA, Iron, Zinc, and more vitamins to support all systems. I sarted doubling Curcumin up to 900 mg and then to 1800 mg of to alleviate the inflammation in my joints caused by the cytokines.

The Alisa Igg and the Western Blot lab tests for Lyme were both negative. No matter my requests, they would not let me see the results of the full Western Blot, which would have supplied important Lyme exposure information. In any case, the Alisa Igg and the Western Blot tests for Lyme were known to be highly inaccurate. The accuracy according to sources is 53%.

I scheduled an appointment with an infectious disease doctor under my health plan. The doctor went over my labs and insisted that I did not have Lyme and even that the photo of the bite mark was not an EM (even though it clearly was). I argued with him that I had four or more clinical symptoms: The EM, the bullesye which I'd photographed, the strange sore throat, the "pins and needles" or "bites from within", the migrating joint pain, and previously sweats and chills.

Again he insisted that I did not have Lyme, that I should not hire a quack and that someday there would be a cure all in the same gulp. I left his office that day devastated. I was aware of the CDC reports stating that without treatment, Lyme disease can spread to a person's heart, joints, and nervous system, causing intense headaches, painful arthritis, facial palsy, and heart palpitations.

For a little while, I started writing letters to his boss. I sent complaints which went nowhere. Then I realized that nothing would be accomplished by doing this. I was wasting my time and life force.

At some point, I tried tinctures from a

homeopath that a family member on the East Coast had recommended since it had worked for her family. This did nothing for me.

I bought two of the most famous books for Lyme. One was for herb treatments. I tried some of the treatments from there. Nothing seemed to work, at least the way I tried it, and in the duration I tried it.

Unlike the established medical community, the "Lyme Healing Community" seemed to be on the same page in their modeling of the Lyme problem. It had recognized that there were three types of Lyme spirochetes' disguises. In the first few days after receiving a bite from an infected tick, doxycycline might be able to knock out the Lyme spirochete. However, Borrelia burgdorferi, the spirochete, a bacteria that causes Lyme disease has a few more disguises once inside its host over longer periods of time. The second form Lyme takes in the body is called persisters which are also known as the round bodies, and the third form are the microcolonies. The persisters and micro-colonies are in a form of drug tolerant dormancy, which means that they will remain dormant, but still alive while the infected person takes medications such as doxycyline and other pharmaceutical cocktails. The last more hidden form Lyme takes is in the plasma, what is known as the Lyme biofilm. The treatment method recommended by one of these texts was to target all of these at once to get rid of Lyme.

What the medical establishment hadn't taken into account in their analysis of fighting Lyme is that the persisters and microcolonies could hide while antibiotic cocktails were in use. When the drug cocktails were no longer in use, the Lyme persisters and microcolonies, would resurface. The medical establishment term for the resurfacing symptoms is "Post-Treatment Lyme Disease Syndrome".

Quickly, I searched for a Lyme-aware doctor

or LAD. The doctor I found suggested that I go on a drip. It would be $600 twice a week, and I did not have that kind of money. I asked what treatments had worked before. This doctor told me that each patient was different and each treatment was unique. I was pretty sure that my case was pure Lyme, that the payload of the tick was completely Lyme since there were no other symptoms to suggest Babesiosis or any of the other myriad Lyme-related infections.

I asked if we could follow an allopathic (oral) treament from Dr Horowitz's book *How Can I Get Better*. The doctor had me take several drugs to target all the forms of Lyme. Almost a year into treatment on December 19, 2018, I started tracking my symptoms with ClickTrack, a phone app which I was using to count as many as 15 symptoms a day, what I was calling internal bites or "pins and needles".

After some time, all my symptoms were diminished by what I would intuitively estimate to be 97%. All the joint pain was gone. There were no other symptoms except what I called the "pins and needles" or being bitten from within.

By January 25, 2020, I was counting four symptoms a day. We tried yet another cocktail from this book. The results were still at 97%. I knew that a common cold would go away at 97%. However, Lyme would not go away, but would be able to repopulate. I knew that just one single Lyme spirochete in the body would be able to repopulate. I was basically treading water in the treatment. This was worthwhile because I was preventing further destruction of my organs. However, Lyme was not going away, not being completely irradicated.

Finally, after learning of Disulfiram (p 21.) from my Lyme-aware doctor, I decided to try it. It took months to get ready, to have the courage to stop the 97% workable yet incomplete antibiotic cocktail.

Researching Lyme

All the researchers of Lyme, as well as their supporters such as the Cohen Foundation are heroes: The Stanford Research Lab, the John Hopkins Lab, the UC and USC Labs, and countless other laboratories, researchers, and doctors including Dr. Kim Lewis, Dist. Professor and the Director of Antimicrobial Discovery Center at Northeastern University, Dr. Ken Liegner and Dr. Daniel A. Kinderlehrer. These and many others are heroes for their countless hours of work to bring out the truth about Lyme and find a cure for so many. To all of them I am grateful.

Online, I spent hours researching Lyme. For your sake, do your research. You'll probably need to, thinking there's got to be some way out of here. Look for the latest research. Go down the rabbit hole. I'm simply leaving you with the straight and narrow of what in the end mattered to me and what saved my life. There are a few important links in the index. Please read these.

If you have the money that someone like Alec Baldwin or Jeff Bridges has, by all means take yourself to the best clinics East or West. If you can do that, you probably don't need this book except as encouragement.

On the Horizon: Hygromycin A

In October 2021, the good news of Hygromycin A, a narrow spectrum antibiotic, was released. Mice were infected with the main Lyme infection of a ticks' payload, the spirochete Borrelia burgdorferi. These mice were cleared of the infection in 5 days with twice a day doses of Hygromycin A. Hygromycin A was also free of toxicity regardless of the dose. Wonderful. It seeems this book might be uneccessary if Hygromycin were available. However, even with the incredible efficacy and what seams like remarkable safety of Hygromycin A, it may be two to three years before the FDA clears it unless there is a push such as there has been with the covid vaccines.

Repurposing Disulfiram

As early as 2016 and prior, a Stanford research team led by Jayakumar Rajadas, PhD, Assistant Professor of Medicine and Director of Stanford's Biomaterials and Advanced Drug Delivery Laboratory, and Research Associate Venkata Raveendra Pothineni, PhD, had been performing high throughput tests on 8000 known substances against all the Lyme forms. There were a few combinations which worked against Lyme; among the top 20 were Azlocillin and Disulfiram.

The Steven and Alexandra Cohen Foundation had established the Cohen Lyme and Tick-borne Disease Initiative, a division within their philanthropic organization focused on supporting Lyme and tick-borne disease research. They have committed to contributing over 60 million dollars toward 25 Lyme disease research projects, Lymedisease.org reported. In 2016, the Cohen Foundation sponsored the first annual "Lyme Disease in the Era of Precision Medicine" conference at the Mount Sinai School of Medicine in New York. At that conference, Dr. Kim Lewis, leader of Northeastern University's Antimicrobial Discovery Center, presented data on the relative effectiveness of different antibiotics against Borrelia burgdorferi, Bb. This he demonstrated in his lab as had Stanford Lab's research. Dr. Lewis had been testing different pharmaceuticals against Bb, and one of the drugs he tested was Disulfiram, also known as "Antabuse". During his talk, Lewis showed a slide in which Disulfiram out-performed the other drug candidates against Borrelia burgdorferi, the culprit for Lyme.

Another drug candidate, Azlocillin, is still on the horizon according to a Standford Medicine News article in March 2020. Azlocillin was effective against the spirochetes and the semi-dormant round bodies. The journal reports that "Pothineni and Rajadas have patented the compound for the treatment of Lyme disease and are working with a company to develop an oral form of the drug". We look forward to hearing more about Azlocillin.

What is Disufiram aka Antabuse

The least costly of the 8000 known substances researched by Standford Lab was Disulfiram. Disulfiram is essentially an old school medicine which is both inexpensive and is able to target cancer. It's main use was to prevent alcoholics from drinking by giving patients painful symptoms after drinking which would require a trip to the hospital for the antidote.

Dr. Ken Liegner of Pawling, NY, learned about Disulfiram, and a willing patient, "Patient Zero" we will call him, offered himself to science. "Interestingly, the patient had had a psychiatric hospitalization during treatment, which he related to significant situational stress. Dr. Liegner was concerned because there have been rare reports of

Disulfiram causing psychiatric problems. The patient did not think these problems had been caused by the drug, and said, "Even if it was responsible, it was worth it! Don't fail to offer it to people just because of that!" The patient continued to be symptom-free over two years later." See reference in index. Daniel A. Kinderlehrer MD learned of Dr Leigner's earliest three patients including Patient Zero and now has 90 patients on Disulfiram. (see reference in index).

The Case for Disulfiram

Here's the case for taking Disulfiram.

1) Disulfiram will protect the biome in contrast to the other allopathic treatments. The biome has been increasingly considered to be central to human health.

2) Disulfiram saves the organs, including the brain, heart, lungs and joints from Lyme.

3) Disulfiram is inexpensive and doesn't require a costly drip.

4) Disulfiram has ended Lyme in various patients.

5) Even if ending Lyme in a patient is not achieved, Disulfiram will limit the damage of Lyme, protecting the patient until Hygromycin A or something else is available.

Starting Disulfiram

I ordered Disulfiram from India in 250 mg tablets, as my LAD suggested. It took a while to arrive and weeks more before I could start taking it. After getting off all the antibiotics--the Flagyll, the Zythromax, whatever, I waited and then started down this path. It was not easy. This is an abridged version of what went down and the things I think are important to learn from my mistakes. There are instructions on how to start up on Disulfiram at half doses. This book doesn't describe how to do that. It will help to check sources such as from Kinderleher (p. 61) and work with your doctor on these approaches.

Backing Off & Finding Balance

When I didn't feel well, I backed off. It could mean backing off Disulfiram, increasing nasal moisture or making sure I had enough water with electrolytes which for me was about 88 to 120 oz per day. In any case, this meant making adjustments until I felt better.

Attitude

Keep positive friends. You'll need every bit of your strength. I stopped watching the news. Online, live resources such as the teachings from His Holiness the Dalai Lama and gazing meditation with Braco really encouraged me. I used EFT tapping for anxiety with Brad Yates. Walking is a great practice to lift one's spirits. Get up every morning knowing you will recover. It may take time to get that attitude. Joel Osteen's positive words may help. He's a Christian theologian who is teaching an uplifting mindset. This was and is important to me in my recovery.

Chinese Medicine (TCM)

It dawned on me that I could get TCM acupuncture and herbs at a local medical school clinic. I treated with them for four or so weeks. This is the powder formula (mostly

cinnamon) that they treated me with which greatly reduced my fear:
Gui Zhi Tong 120 grams
Gui Zhi 20 grams
Long Gu 25 grams
Mu Li 25 grams.

Chocolate & Caffeine

I wasn't eating much chocolate to begin with. When I did, these were my top choices for relatively low sugar chocolate:

◊ Alter Eco 90% Cacao Mint Blackout
◊ Nib Mor Organic Dark Chocolate 72% Cacao with Dark Cherry
◊ Trader Joe's Uganda 85% Dark Chocolate Bar
◊ Power Crunch Chocolate

Some people don't think you should drink caffeine because of an interaction with Disulfiram, which I also noticed. Due to this interaction, I only use a splash of coffee with milk and hot water, none at all, decaf green tea with ginger or an entire cup of oolong tea. (see page 25.)

The Dose

We decided to take Disulfiram as one dose per day to apply direct pressure to the spirochetes at once and not split the dose.

Drinking Liquids & No Alcohol

It is really important to reiterate that Disulfiram is not to be taken with alcohol or fermented products, even vinegar, Kumbucha or Probiotic 1% drinks. It was no trouble for me to not drink alcohol. My total daily intake of liquids was about 88 to 108 oz per day with electrolytes. I drank water with several packets of Ultima Replenisher in a 40 oz bottle with a half teaspoon of CALM in the first 40 oz. To make sure I was getting enough calcium, I drank Trader Joe's or Clover Organic 1% Milk which also has more potassium than both whole milk and low fat. Later, I started using Magnesium Glycinate capsules instead of CALM because CALM taken together with Disulfiram can result in softening of the stools. Coffee seemed to have a bit of an electric interaction with

Disulfiram, so I eventually reduced coffee to just a splash. I wanted my liquids, including milk or a light splash of coffee over milk and hot water to add up to about 88-120 oz per day. I sometimes didn't reach this target which meant the next day was in part a make up, that is, drinking more to make up for it. A sweet amount of liquid hovered around 104 oz which meant clearer sinuses and perhaps less headaches since this flushed my system.

Water electrolytes to add to water:
◊ Ultima Replenisher in Raspberry
◊ Nuun Hydration Tangerine Lime

Here are some high potassium drinks I liked:
◊ Columbia Gorge Organic
Plant-Based Nutrition
◊ Real-Pressed Carrot Beet Celery
◊ Real-Pressed JUST GREENS
◊ Biotto Organic Beet Juice
◊ Trader Joe's Organic Green Juice

Dairy

◊ Trader Joe's 1% Organic Milk
◊ Organic Clover 1% Milk
◊ Horizon Organic Milk DHA Omega-3
◊ Red Hill Farm Goak Milk Kefir
◊ Trader Joe's Goat Milk Kefir

Drugs

In my case, I was not taking any other prescribed drugs. I very occasionally used chewable low dose aspirin orange flavor. Before Lyme, I hardly had any headaches at all. After I got Lyme, most of my headaches seemed to be due to dry sinuses and what I see as dehydration while taking Disulfiram. However, I discovered a much longer list of other causes which is in the section on headaches.

Immodium. In nearly a middle stretch of treatment there were about 12 days when I forgot to take my vitamins, causing me to have a bad case of diarrhea. Yes, I caved and took four Immodiums in one day when

I forgot to keep up on vitamins and follow up with probiotics. Never do this, okay?

Here are my alternative medicines:
◊ Plum Flower Pe Min Kan Wan to knock out a sinus cold
◊ Similasan Sinus (or Allergy) Relief spray
◊ Allergy Releaf System for allergies
◊ Plantiva AllerDX for allergies
◊ Boiron Sinus Calm
◊ Qing Qi Hua Tan Wan powder to knock out a lung cold
◊ Zyrtec for allergy relief when I was desperate to stop blowing my nose.

Entertainment

I wanted the lightest entertainment I could get, such as watching the Warriors play basketball. I turned the news down to the lowest tolerable level, which was late night and some online news. I suggest turning this off as much as you are able. Don't worry, your friends won't notice and the news will get to you anyway. Watch uplifting movies instead.

Environment

Where I live the air is sometimes dry. I bought a Hessaire MC18M evaporative cooler. It runs about $135-150. (To dry it out after use, set it as just a fan for 30 minutes. I would clean it out periodically by adding one cup of white cider vinegar or hydrogen peroxide.) I ran it in stretches when it seemed like the air had dried out. This helped with the dry air headaches I would get. What I mean here is my sinuses would dry out and I would get headaches. Now, I believe that more hydration while treating with Disulfiram, up to 104 oz per day, also helped maintain moisture in the sinuses. These headaches seemed to go away entirely from the multipronged approaches I followed, including Similasan Sinus Relief spray and a 9 x 13 pan of water near my bed in addition to the hydration.

Exercise

It will keep you happier if you keep exercising. During stetches, I walked three miles or more per day. Sometimes I was doing up to six miles and sometimes less. Later I was on a stationary bicycle. During covid, I dropped my gym membership. I also used 3 pound weights on the upper body and core exercises. Find something you can do which you will enjoy. Yes to dancing even in your kitchen or living room. A stationary bicyling if it's raining or running interval training is good if you like doing this. Use a quarter mile track and run one quarter and walk two quarters of the track and then continue to alternate running another quarter track and walking two quarters. Your system will still be elevated while you are just walking.

Missing a day of exercise is a day we don't get to redo. Yes, and I too miss some.

Just do it, Zen Master Seung Sahn said.

Foods

In my case I mostly limited bread in sandwhiches and corn tortillas while still eating the contents of a yummy taco.

Here are some foods I enjoyed:

◊ Tera's Whey Grass Fed Organic Whey Protein Unsweetened

◊ Tera's Whey Grass Fed Organic Whey Protein Organic Bourbon Vanilla

◊ Orgain Organic Protein Plant Based Protein Powder

◊ Casa Sanchez Mild Tomate Verde Salsa

◊ Casa Sanchez Real Guacamole

Foods (continued)

Trader Joe's Products

◊ Old Fashioned Rolled Oats

◊ Chia seeds

◊ Himalayan Salt

◊ Chimichurri Rice with frozen vegetables

◊ Fresh Harvest Petite Peas frozen

◊ Spicy Jalapeño Chicken Sausage

also in Garlic Herb, Spicy Italian or Pesto

◊ Bilinski's Chicken Saugage, Cilantro Lime

◊ Organic Carrots

◊ Blueberries

◊ Grapefruit

◊ Organic Triple Filtered Coconut Oil

◊ Trader Joe's Mixed Organic Greens

◊ Organic Kale

◊ Organic Swiss Chard or Rainbow Chard

◊ Trader Joe's Lentil Soup (canned)

Friends

Family and a few other people on earth besides doctors in the San Francisco Bay Area knew I had Lyme. Let's face it, you'll want people who can keep your secret if you are in stealth mode. There are friends of mine whom I've told I have Lyme. Two of them won't believe that I have Lyme without positive lab tests. All of them are keeping my secret as far as I know.

Headaches

Before Lyme, I hardly had any headaches at all. During Lyme treatment, I discovered nine kinds of headaches. One is a salt headache from too much salt, one is a headache from not enough liquid, the third is a herx, which is the die off of spirochetes, which I will describe in the next section. The fourth is a TMJ headache, the fifth is a sinus headache from dried out sinuses, the sixth headache is due to not enough sleep, the seventh could be stopping coffee if you do that, the eighth is a headache from a lack of electrolytes. The ninth is a headache from not enough Vitamin K2, which you can get by eating greens and red meats, such as lamb. Wow, from no headaches hardly ever to nine types of headaches to discern. Remember that I did not have the highest load of spirochetes because I was already at at an estimated 97% resolved symptoms. Besides herxing reactions, most of my headaches were due to dried out sinuses and dehydration. Fragile sinus capillaries are linked to vitamin K2 deficiency. At times, headaches were also caused by a lack electrolytes. In fact, I had an onset of a bad headache. My regular doctor scheduled an MRI and other tests. It turns out I was lacking in chloride which I corrected easily by doubling up on electrolytes.

Herxing aka Herx reaction

According to WhatisLyme.com, "The Jarisch-Herxheimer Reaction, or more commonly known as a "herx," or "herxing" is a detoxification reaction the body has from die off of bacteria.

"As the body detoxifies, or tries to get rid of dead bacteria and toxins, it is not uncommon to experience flu-like symptoms including headache, joint and muscle pain, body aches, sore throat, general malaise, sweating, chills, fever, nausea, hives or other symptoms. This is a normal reaction when starting a treatment for Lyme disease. It indicates that...pathogens are being effectively killed off."

"The Herxheimer Reaction is an immune system reaction to the toxins that are released when large amounts of pathogens are being killed off, and the body does not eliminate the toxins quickly enough. Simply stated, it is a reaction that occurs when the body is detoxifying and the released toxins, (endotoxins) are released from the cell walls of dying bacteria [which is] due to effective treatment... The important thing to note is that worsening symptoms do not indicate failure of the treatment in question; in fact, usually just the opposite." In my case, my herxing amounted to headaches which I go into in the previous section on headaches. Drinking plenty of water with electrolytes Vitamin C, nicotinamide, selenium and N-acetyl cysteine (NAC) and Glutathione will help prevent and clear Herx reactions.

How I took Disulfiram

Taking Disulfiram with some food is the way to go. Practically, I have an iron stomache. For two years I was on cocktails of antibiotics and the only thing which bothered me was flagyll. This is because I was able to support the biome with probiotics. I would eat something with Disulfiram. Since I would usually take the Disulfiram sometime after dinner, I took it with something like a granny smith apple and or a splash of milk or snack.

Intensity

When I found myself feeling intense, I

checked my blood pressure, but it wasn't that. It was a lack of calcium and magnesium. I cut my coffee intake down to a splash of coffee with hot water or none at all. Milk lightened the sense of intensity I was feeling. and I also adopted Magnesium Glycinate.

Keeping Stools Firm

Sometimes, I paused CALM because of softening stools, although it is a great product. Eating veggies with meat or lentils and rice with veggies also helped keep stools firm.

Liver Labs & Lyme Tests

When I was taking the allopathic antibiotic combinations over a period of two years, RBC and liver panels were a must. High liver labs, ie ALT and AST, could be lowered in a week or two, or a month with two capsules of Beet Powder Root per day and regular exercise. (I have the labs to prove this). Lyme tests were negative, and yet I knew I had

Lyme. These tests for Lyme were known to be highly inaccurate. I was left with the option of spending thousands on more accurate tests to prove I had Lyme, which I knew I had, or get treatment without proving I had Lyme with more lab tests.

Logging & Record Keeping

I used ClickTrack, an Iphone app, when I was counting symptoms early on to count the "pins and needles' or bites. Later I used Google sheets to track medicine intake and symptoms. In the first column was the dose, the next the date and time I took it, the next column the number of hours between doses, and the next column contained the liquids for the day including ounces of milk, ginger or green tea, and here I also listed "vitamins". In the last column, I described any symptoms, feelings or whatever would be helpful to sort things out.

Keeping a regular journal is a lot harder than I ever imagined. Although I got better at this, there were days that I had to fill in, guessing some of the details of the day before. This Google sheet was not a food journal. Some people might want to keep a food journal if their foods are not in the safe zone. By safe, I mean they are known and they aren't cause for digestive concern.

Losing the contents of the bowels

Surprise. Expulsion of the contents of my intestines, accompanied with hiding that while trying to get back to my car and home was new to me. This was Not Pretty - and required showering up along with washing clothes.

If you don't want to lose your bowels, don't take Disulfiram before you have finished all or 97% of the liquids for the day. I had never lost my bowels before this. It's embarrassing and I was just lucky I had a Patagonia jacket that I could tie around my waist to hide the collatoral damage. One time, I was on a solo walk in the early evening and had to quickly return to the car and race home.

Another time, I'd taken a whole bunch of vitamins and drank 40 oz of water in the car. I was desperate to find the loo. I made it to a Whole Foods and had to run back to my car, luckily I had a jacket to tie around my waist. These lessons happened and I regrouped to realize what was going on. Just in case, you might want to have spare clothes for an emergency. I was not prepared.

Repeating this: If I didn't want to lose my bowels, I learned to take Disulfiram sometime after finishing all of the liquids for the day.

Lyme vs Lyme Disease

This was essential for me: I did not talk about Lyme very much and did not refer to what I had as Lyme disease. I did not want to see myself as having a disease, just a visitor. I did not want this to be my life identity or direction.

Meals

Breakfast

Trader Joe's Old Fashioned Rolled Oats with banana or raisins. Hard boiled eggs or scrambled eggs with dash of goat kefir.

Breakfast, Snack, or Dessert

One scoop whey powder over Trader Joe's frozen fruit and a 1/2 to 3/4 cups of kefir or yogurt.

Lunch

Your call. I liked these frozen Amy's dishes:

◊ Harvest Casserole Bowl

◊ Indian Vegetable Korma Curried Vegetables with Dal

◊ Blackeyed Peas and Veggies

If you live in the San Francisco Bay Area, Poulet in Berkeley has delicious Raw Kale Salad and Rosemary Lemon Chicken Breast or Legs-- it is the best dinner in town for just over ten dollars. Wow, to their fantastic Carrot Cake!

Dinner Dish A

As mainly a fish, turkey or lamb eater, I ate lamb about every three weeks and sometimes less after the headaches were not a thing. Lentils and Rice with two globs of coconut oil, lemon and Himalayan salt is a soothing dish to eat and then store in the fridge. On another day, I would add greens such as kale, brocolli and swiss chard. Himalayan salt will make anything taste great.

Dinner Dish B

Trader Joe's Chimichurri Rice with Trader Joe's Fresh Harvest Petite Peas (the organic one's are sometimes too pasty). I add a meat to this. I use Trader Joe's Spicy Jalapeño Chicken Sausage which also comes in Garlic Herb and Spicy Italian or Bilinski's Chicken Saugage, Cilantro Lime and also add Trader Joe's Power Greens.

Meditation

Practicing meditation will help you feel lighter as you learn the practice of letting go of thoughts. Let go of any frustration you encounter as soon as you create it as if it is a hot stove. An even temperament will be a great result if you keep up a practice.

Nix the News

It's up to you. What's going on in the world is really important to me. However, I'm on somewhat of a break to protect my well-being. I honor those whose job it is (and it is all of our jobs) to protect our country. All the news you need to hear will come to you.

Nose

Cleaning out my nose on a daily basis is important because breathing is important. I want to remove any obstruction to breathing. The phlegm, mucus or snot is the body's attempt to clear away pathogens.

Pain

Early on, I took 1800 mg of curcumin for the pain in my joints caused by inflammatory cytokines. The pain had reached 8-9 out of 10. Curcumin reduced and ended my pain along with the alliopathic treatment. It also acts as a blood thinner, so be aware and check with a doctor if you are on these.

Probiotics

The goal is to keep your biome healthy. Taking probiotics an hour after taking Disulfiram is a good idea. I realized this late in the game and because I was often already in bed by that time, I wasn't doing this myself. However, it also works to have it in the day's vitamin haul.

Here's a great probiotic at a good price which does not require refrigeration:
New Rhythm Probiotics 20 Strains 50 Billion CFU. I take 1-2 capsules per day. Again, this is also welcome in your daily vitamins.

There's nothing wrong with keeping the biome stoked with plenty of probiotics. I believe this assists in preventing loose stools.

Products which worked for me

It's imperative to avoid products with alcohols. Generally, the names of these products end in "ol". I was already avoiding ethylene glycol. I was able to use natural soaps. I researched these from various lists from others and I tested others myself.

◊ Similasan Sinus (or Allergy) Relief spray
◊ Burt's Bees Pomegranate
◊ Alba Even Advanced Daily Cream
◊ Cerave Daily Moisturizing Lotion
◊ Dr Bronner's 4-in-1 Peppermint Organic Sugar Soap
◊ EO Essential Oils Organic Hand sanitizer was okay for me to use.
◊ Jason Sea Fresh Antiplaque & Strengthening Paste Deep Sea Spearmint
◊ Neutrogena Naturals Purifying Facial Cleanser

◊ Puracy Natural Children's Body Wash
◊ Trader Joe's Nourish Spa Shampoo
◊ Trader Joe's Nourish Antioxident Facial Serum
◊ Trader Joe's Shea Butter & Coconut Oil Hair Mask
◊ Carapex Elastin & Collagen day cream
◊ Eva Hyaluronic Acid Serum

Showers

Take showers at least two or three times a week. A bath on Sunday night is good. These will help lift your spirits. You will also breathe better since the moisture will help clear out your sinuses.

Skin

Lotions, chapstick and facial cleansers may have alcohol or alcohol derivates in them. Be careful of these as they may create an unpleasant stinging or full-blown headache. If the dose is really high, it could trigger a reaction with Disulfiram and send you to the hospital. I made a habit of reading all the ingredients before buying a product. One time, however, I did get a sudden headache after I bought a new lip balm. I didn't know if that was what had caused the headache, but I decided to wait on using it again.

Sleep

The body needs sleep to repair and defend itself. Sleep also improves well-being. Getting sleep is a priority for me.

Snacks

I tried making my own popcorn and just didn't like cleaning up after it even though I was good at making it. Here are my go to snacks (along with Chocolates listed on p. 23).

◊ Almonds
◊ Pecans
◊ Walnuts
◊ Raisins
◊ Equadoran Organic Bananas
◊ Organic Cellery (wish I'd done more)
◊ Trader Joe's Raw Organic Green Beans
◊ Trader Joe's Organic Cut & Peeled Carrots
◊ Trader Joe's Mediterranean Hummus
◊ Trader Joe's Smooth & Creamy Roasted

Red Pepper Hummus
◊ The Hummus Guy Spanish Artichoke
Flat Parsley Sprouted Hummus
◊ gimMe Organic Roasted Seaweed
◊ Trader Joe's Persian Cucumbers
◊ Trader Joe's Granny Smith Apples
◊ Mission Organic Blue Corn Tortilla Chips
◊ Trader Joe's Organic Salted Popcorn [Fav]
◊ Lesser Evil Organic Popcorn
◊ Whole Foods Organic Classic Popcorn

Sweets

Already I was avoiding sugar for the most part. The general wisdom is to avoid sugar since the spirochetes thrive on it, so I very rarely ate any cake, except an excellent Carrot Cake from Poulet in Berkeley.

Also, I rarely ate ice cream. My favorite flavors are Haagen-Dazs Bourbon Vanilla or Mint Chip or Breyer's Mint Chip. The pies I bought for events were Berry Supreme by Upper Crust or Whole Foods' Lime Berry Pie. Eating cookies was not a thing for me, or so I thought until I found out that Lavender

Bakery & Cafe in Berkeley has oatmeal chocolate chip cookies.

Symptom Corrections or Disambiguations

I thought I was getting headaches from a lack of red meat, though they could also have been caused by a lack of leafy greens. They could also have resulted from a lack of electolytes, dehydration or dry air. On one occasion I had a sudden onset of a bad headache. It turns out that I was lacking in chloride which was simply corrected by adding more electrolytes. Lamb and other red meats, as well as the leafy greens increase Vitamin K which helps to mend the sinus capillaries dammaged in dyhrdation. Also, physical intensity, a kind of squirming in the body, was linked to a lack of calcium and magnesium. During this time, I started taking Magnesium Glycinate. The Disulfiram regimen together with the visiting spirochetes were affecting my body in a whole lot of ways that required more focus than what is normally required in day to day life.

Teeth

When my teeth got sensitive I realized it was a sign that I was not getting enough calcium. Later in the game, I just resolved to drink enough milk to be sure I was getting enough calcium. How much was enough? I looked it up. The WHO said 500 mg and the UK says 700 mg. To recover from being calcium deficient, I decided to drink mulptiple quarts of milk per day until I felt it was resolved. It was definitely more than I needed, so afterward, I decided to drink two cups of 1% organic milk, providing 780 mg of calcium per day.

Vitamins & Liquids

Forgetting to take my vitamins, even though it was listed in my Google sheet, and not getting enough calcium for 14 days imbalanced my system. How can you do this you ask with a spreadsheet? I think you'll be surprised how easy it is to lose track even when you are tracking.

The best time I found for taking vitamins is during the day before or between drinking courses of liquid. It's estimated that 20 oz an hour may be properly absorbed by the body per hour. The total intake for liquids could be water with electrolytes, it could be 16 oz of oolong tea, two- eight oz of milk with eight ounces of water with the total hovering around 104 oz. To keep track of liquids, the forty ounce Klean Kanteens of water with 2 packets of Ultima Raspberry, taken twice a day are great. It's best to take the vitamins a good deal away from Disulfiram. Suffice it to say that taking vitamins near Disulfiram caused a disasterous explosion for me in my gut which resulted in a race to the john and we don't want that for you.

The spirochetes feed on some of the same nutrients our bodies need. Sometimes, I took a break from eating all these vitamins and hand selected just a few of them.

Vitamins or Supplements I'm regularly taking:
◊ B 50, NOW
◊ Complete Omega, Nordic Naturals
◊ Vitamin D3 5000 iu, NOW
◊ Super Bio Vitamin C, Soloray
◊ Bio Zinc, Soloray
◊ B6 Folic Acid, B12 Trader Joe's
◊ K2 500 mcg, Superior Source
◊ NAC, 600 mg, NOW
◊ Alpha Lypoic Acid, 600 mg, Nutricost
◊ Glutathione, 500 mg, NOW (for Herx Reactions)
◊ E-400, NOW
◊ L-Arginine, 500 mg, Amazing Formulas
◊ Iron 18 mg NOW
◊ Hyaluronic Acid, 100 mg, NO
◊ Astaxanthin from microalgae, SR
◊ Nattokinase, 4000 FU, 200 or 500 mg (for the plasma/biofilm form of spirochete)

Probiotics:
◊ New Rhythm 20 Strains 50 Bn cfu
◊ Physician's Choice Probiotic 60 Bn

Pain:
◊ Turmeric Curcumin 500 mg, Puritan's Pride (to reduce inflammation from cytokines)

Liver Support:
◊ LiveBlend SP-13 475 mg, Soloray or
◊ Milk Thistle, Jarrow Formulas
◊ Beet Root, 1000 mg, Nature's Way

Magnesium and Calcium:
◊ Magnesium Glycinate, Pharmaca, 400 mg or
◊ CALM 1 teaspoon in 40 oz of water if stools are remaining firm
◊ Clover or Trader Joe's Milk Organic 1%
◊ Bone Up, Jarrow Formulas
◊ Collagen Type I & III, NeoCell (Spirochetes damage collagen)
◊ Iron 18 mg NOW

Kidneys:
◊ Kidney Cleanse, Sunergetic

Here's what I took sporadically:
◊ CoQ1-0 400 mg
◊ DHM, 300 mg Pure Nootropics
◊ DHM 1000, Double Wood (I never really figured these two out)
◊ Ginger, 1000 mg, Wild Harvest
◊ Palmetto, 580 mg, Soloray

Weight

Some people gain weight on Disulfiram. In my case, I ate only two meals a day plus snacks. I lost 13 pounds in my last year of Lyme. I also exercised by walking, dancing, stationary bicycling and sometimes working on core body exercises. To weigh myself, I did this naked before eating and starting the day.

Most Important Antabuse Secrets I followed.

1. Breakfast: Eating Trader Joe's Rolled Oats, sometimes with eggs or another other protein.
2. Taking vitamins before or between first and second 40 oz of water. Using two 40 oz. Klean Kanteens was one way which helped keep to track of water intake with electrolytes. I resolved to never take vitamins near Disulfiram unless I wanted a mess to clean up. Use your imagination.
3. Drinking liquid in stages during the late morning and during the afternoon into early evening ending around 7:30 PM. Usually 88-120 oz per day and hovering around 104 oz per day was ideal for sinus moisture and a lack of headaches.
4. To water I added two packets of Raspberry Ultima in each of the 40 ozs of water. Ultima comes in 20 individual packages. Raspberry was the flavor I preferred. See page 52.
5. I took Disulfiram after I had finished the water for the day (6:30-7:30) so as not to lose the bowels.
6. I aimed to take my appropriate weight dose of 250 mg of Disulfiram at 9:15 PM plus or minus about an hour.

7. Taking Disulfiram with food-- eating it with a Granny Smith apple or milk. I had an iron stomache. Eat something with Disulfiram. I also learned to float the medicine down my throat so it would not to stick to the back of my throat.
8. Taking 2 Priobiotics an hour after taking Disulfiram to protect the biome. I used New Rhythm Probiotics 20 Strains 50 Billion CFU. I didn't remember to do this as much as I would have liked. (It's in daily vitamins, too.)
9. Getting a good 8 hours of sleep. How are you going to recover without it? I started to go to bed at an earlier time, 10:00 PM.
10. I repeat, I learned not to take vitamins near Disulfiram, for me it was not pretty.
11. Keeping a Google sheet to keep records. Set up with these columns of dose, date and time, liquids and vitamins, issues. Keeping a regular journal in the last column is an important support to see how we are doing and sleuthing out changes we might need.
12. Drinking liquids: milk and water, ginger tea with CALM, water and electrolytes.

POSTFACE

Dear Readers,

On 2/22/22 in a moment of synchronicity, I attended a Harvard webinar with Kris Newby producer of the documentary, *Under the Skin*, and award-winning journalist Brian Owens author of *Lyme Disease in Canada.*

Kris Newby and her husband contracted Lyme in 2002 while on Martha's Vineyard. She said it took 5 years, 10 doctors and $60,000 to finally get her disease under control. Kris produced the award-winnging documentary *Under the Skin* and her book *Bitten* has won three international book awards.

The award-winning documentary shows the harrowing pain of people infected with Lyme. It estimates the pandemic number of Lyme patients in the US, eclipsing the numbers of both those with HIV and breast cancer.

Remembering this incredible suffering around the world, it is my deepest wish that this book offers people a way to recover from Lyme until better methods such as Hydromycin A becomes available. Godspeed.

> It is my deep wish that you or a loved one or friend soon recovers from Lyme. May it be soon.

Remember everything there is to be grateful for.

Take it from His Holiness the Dalai Lama,
"Never give up."[1]

Don't ever forget you are unique and you are here for a reason. Remember that.

Sending blessings your way,

Fonda Living

March 31, 2022

[1] His Holiness the 14th Dalai Lama.

INDEX

I spent hours researching Lyme. If you saw every reference, it would be overwhelming for you and for me. I'm simply leaving you with the straight and narrow of what in the end mattered to save my life. The list is in no particular order.

Disulfiram–breakthrough drug for Lyme and other tick-borne diseases? By Daniel A. Kinderlehrer MD
"A patient of Dr. Ken Liegner of Pawling, New York, saw the lecture by Dr. Kim Lewis on YouTube and asked to be treated with disulfiram."
https://www.lymedisease.org/disulfiram-kinderlehrer/

"Ninety of my patients are now on disulfiram... "I suggest starting with low doses, 62.5 mg or 125 mg every three days. Vitamin C, nicotinamide, selenium and N-acetyl cysteine (NAC) will help prevent Herx reactions
https://www.lymedisease.org/disulfiram-kinderlehrer-2/

Azlocillin
Lyme Disease Bacteria Eradicated by New Drug in Early Tests by Kris Newby
https://scopeblog.stanford.edu/2020/03/30/lyme-disease-bacteria-eradicated-by-new-drug-in-early-tests/

"In 2016, Venkata Raveendra Pothineni and colleagues at Stanford reported on new drug candidates against Borrelia burgdorferi, Bb, using a technique known as high-throughput screening. They ranked disulfiram as number one in activity against Bb among their top 20 hits."
https://www.lymedisease.org/disulfiram-kinderlehrer/

Hydromycin A
Drug treatment for Lyme disease could lead to its eradication, by Michael Le Page
https://www.newscientist.com/article/2292543-drug-treatment-for-lyme-disease-could-lead-to-its-eradication/
[Hygromycin A,] A selective antibiotic for Lyme disease
https://www.sciencedirect.com/science/article/abs/pii/S0092867421010588

Metamorphoses of Lyme disease spirochetes: phenomenon of Borrelia persisters
https://www.ncbi.nlm.nih.gov/pmc/articles/PMC6521364/

Dr Richard I Horowitz's book, How Can I Get Better, An Action Plan for Treating Resistant Lyme and Chronic Disease
https://www.youtube.com/watch?v=92pi2RoSYz8&ab_channel=FriendsHealthConnection

Dr. Kim Lewis, PhD, co-founder of NovoBiotic Pharmaceuticals, Developing Therapies for Lyme Disease, 2021 LDA CME Conf.
https://www.youtube.com/watch?v=BolFS1VE3eA&ab_channel=LymeDiseaseAssociation%2CInc.

https://lymediseaseassociation.org/lda-conferences/lda-conf-2021/2021-faculty-bios-talk-summaries/kim-lewis-phd/

Award-winning Documentary,
Under Our Skin films
https://underourskin.com/uos1#film
https://underourskin.com/emergence

Kris Newby, Producer.

Nev Zubcevik, Chief Medical Officer.
https://www.hack.invisible.international/

Lyme Disease in Canada, award-winning journalist, Brian Owens.

Lyme General Symptom Questionaire
https://www.frontiersin.org/articles/10.3389/fmed.2019.00283/full

Disulfiram for Lyme disease: profiles of two patients reporting good outcomes
by Jennifer Shea
https://www.lymedisease.org/shea-disulfiram-lyme-disease

YOUR NOTES:

Made in United States
North Haven, CT
04 November 2026

21770191R00049